MENIERE'S DISEASE

What is Meniere's, Symptoms, Treatment, and Lifestyle

Pierre Mouchette, author

Life-Health Media USA
An Enviro | Life Knowledge Publication
a subsidiary of Real Property Experts LLC

Copyright © 2021 by Pierre Mouchette

All rights are reserved. No part of this publication may be reproduced, distributed, or transmitted in any form or by any means, including photocopying, recording, or other electronic or mechanical methods, without the prior written permission of the publisher, except in the case of brief quotations embodied in critical reviews and specific other noncommercial uses permitted by copyright law.

ISBN 979-8401885739 (Paperback Book)

Independently Published

First Edition: January 2022
Life-Health Media USA
Web Address: https://www.enviro-life-media.com
Contact: publications@synchronicity-investor.com

Note: This publication comes in various formats, such as Paperbacks and Electronic Books (e-books). Particular material in the paperback version of this book may not be included in e-books, and vice versa.

At Life-Health Media USA, we pride ourselves on every publication's quality, research, and transparency.

Disclaimer

This Life-Health Media USA publication provides information about the subject matter covered. The author and publisher of this content are not acting as healthcare professionals to present covered material. The information and statements are educational and not a substitute for informed medical advice. Do not take any action before consulting a healthcare professional. You are solely responsible for the use of any content. You hold Life-Health Media USA and its members harmless in any event or claim, demand, or damage, including reasonable attorneys' fees, asserted by any third party, or arising out of your use of, or conduct on, this publication and products mentioned.

Life-Health Media USA writers provide applicable content and break down complex topics so they are easier to understand. Information given may not apply to your specific situation, and products or services recommended may not be a good fit for your application. While Life-Health Media USA strives to provide accurate, up-to-date content, we cannot guarantee the accuracy and completeness of the information supplied. By using this content, you understand that all material is an expression of opinion and not professional advice.

The contents of this publication were developed through the writings of licensed and non-licensed medical professionals and other external contributors and are for informational purposes only. The content herein is not a substitute for professional medical advice, diagnosis, or treatment. Always consult your doctor or other qualified healthcare providers with any questions regarding a medical condition, procedure, or treatment. Whether a prescription medication, over-the-counter medicine, vitamin, supplement, or herbal alternative, your physician should review all drugs before purchase or use.

Life-Health Media USA makes no guarantees about the efficiency or safety of products or treatments described in its content. Health conditions and drug information are subject to change and do not include all applications, instructions, precautions, warnings, drug interactions, allergic reactions, or adverse effects.

Life-Health Media USA does not recommend or endorse any specific test, clinician, clinical care provider, product, procedure, opinion, or service mentioned in Life-Health Media USA publications. This publication is not a substitute for informed medical advice, and you should not take any action before consulting with your healthcare provider.

Quality Of Life

Quality of Life (QoL) is a highly subjective measurement essential to the individual's well-being. Factors that play a significant role vary according to personal preferences but usually include financial security, job satisfaction, interpersonal relationships, life-work balance, family life, health, healthy food, safety, and access to cultural and leisure activities.

This publication focuses on HEALTH, that is, the QoL of those affected by this disease. Here we explain in an easy-to-read and understand method 'What is Meniere's, its Symptoms, available Treatment, and Lifestyle.' The reader will utilize the information to help them understand the disease more fully, relieve symptoms, understand treatments, and how lifestyle affects them. Information given will help the reader effectively eliminate the devastating long-term impact of Meniere's disease, thereby enhancing their Quality of Life.

Contents

Part 1   **MENIERE'S DISEASE** .... - 7 -
    What Is Meniere's Disease .... - 7 -
    What Causes Meniere's Disease? .... - 8 -
    Why Are People Who Have Meniere's Always So Fatigued? ..... - 8 -

Part 2   **SYMPTOMS OF MENIERE'S DISEASE** .... - 10 -
    Additional Symptoms of Meniere's Disease .... - 11 -
    The Upper Cervical Solution for Meniere's and Vertigo .... - 11 -
    Damage Caused By Meniere's Disease .... - 12 -

Part 3   **DIAGNOSING MENIERE'S DISEASE** .... - 13 -
    What Type Of Doctor Diagnoses Meniere's? .... - 13 -
    Testing For Meniere's Disease .... - 13 -

Part 4   **TREATMENT OF MENIERE'S DISEASE** .... - 15 -
    Noninvasive Therapies And Procedures .... - 15 -
    Aggressive Procedures .... - 15 -

Part 5   **DIET and MENIERE'S** .... - 17 -
    Diet Goals .... - 17 -
    The Diet .... - 17 -
    Food And Drink To Consume .... - 20 -
    Effectiveness Of The Diet .... - 20 -

Part 6   **VITAMINS, MEDICATIONS, and HERBALS** .... - 21 -
    Over the Counter (OTC) Medications .... - 22 -
    Herbal Treatment Options .... - 23 -

Part 7   **LIFESTYLE CHANGES** .... - 25 -

Part 8   **MISCELLANEOUS SUGGESTIONS** .... - 27 -

Part 9   **CAREGIVERS MANAGEMENT** .... - 29 -

Part 1 MENIERE'S DISEASE

What Is Meniere's Disease

This disease is a chronic disorder of the inner ear. While uncomfortable and disruptive to the quality of life, it is not fatal. All symptoms are associated with dysfunction in the organs of the inner ear, which is responsible for hearing and balance.

Meniere's disease is characterized by four prominent symptoms which occur with varying degrees of intensity:

- **Aural fullness** - a feeling of fullness in the ear, which can be a very bothersome condition that can affect your overall quality of life if left untreated. It could be defined as a sensation of pressure in the ear and muted hearing, pain, itching, drainage, ringing in the ears, and the symptoms of vertigo.

- **Hearing loss** - the degree of hearing loss may range from mild to severe and is typically in one ear but can occur in both. Fluctuating low-frequency sensorineural hearing loss becomes worse during attacks, and hearing may permanently deteriorate over time. Hearing loss, in conjunction with dizziness, makes the disease distressing.

- **Tinnitus** - a ringing or buzzing sound within the ears. The sound may vary in frequency and volume and can occur in either one or both ears. Often, treating underlying conditions can help to lessen the effects of tinnitus. The noise can become very bothersome and interfere with the individual's quality of life. Often, the sound can come and go and will vary in intensity.

- **Vertigo** - a disorder caused by problems within the ear. It may be described as extreme dizziness that makes it seem like the surroundings are moving. This condition can lead to a loss of balance, an upset stomach, vomiting, and nausea. Other symptoms can include jerking movements in the eyes, pain in the head, and ringing or buzzing in the ears, known as tinnitus.
  Note: balance issues become a significant problem because the sensory cells are responsible for balance. To maintain balance, the vestibular system works with your vision to keep objects in focus, and inner ear problems disrupt this process.

Facts about Meniere's disease include:

- In approximately 5% of Meniere's disease cases, there is a positive family history for the condition indicating a genetic component in individuals with Meniere's disease.

- Meniere's disease most frequently affects adults between the ages of 40 to 60. Isolated symptoms can appear between the ages of 20 and 60. It is unusual for people older than 60 to develop the disease.

- Most cases of Meniere's disease are unilateral, where 10 to 50% of people also develop symptoms in the opposite ear.

- Almost 3% of people diagnosed with Meniere's disease are children.

- The male to female ratio of people getting Meniere's will vary from equal to a slight preponderance of females over males. Some women report improvement of symptoms after pregnancy.

- There is no predominance of hearing problems in the right or left ear.

What Causes Meniere's Disease?

The source of this disease is still unknown. But some scientists believe the disease is caused by changes in the fluid of the tubes in the inner ear, whereas others suggest autoimmune disease, allergies, and genetics.

Unusual amounts of fluid (endolymph) in the inner ear include:

- abnormal immune response
- genetic predisposition
- improper fluid drainage, perhaps because of a blockage or anatomic abnormality
- viral infection

Note: an inner ear fluid imbalance affects hearing and balance. The inner ear fluid helps signal your place and space to the brain. For someone with Meniere's, fluid builds up and creates inaccurate messages.

Why Are People Who Have Meniere's Always So Fatigued?

One of the suspected reasons is that the brain receives continuous conflicting information from the damaged balance organ in the inner ear(s) and other components of the balance system, the eyes, and the muscles. In some ways, both the brain and the muscles constantly adjust for the frequently conflicting information, which will wear you out.

The emotional aspect has to do with the constant fatigue to a certain extent. Fatigue makes you need to rest a lot, and as a result, you do not accomplish what you want to, leaving you feeling guilty. Fatigue can also be an indication of depression.

Part 2   SYMPTOMS OF MENIERE'S DISEASE

Meniere's disease's symptoms tend to come on as **episodes** or **attacks.**

Symptoms include:

- aural fullness, or feeling that the ear is full or plugged
- headaches
- loss of balance
- loss of hearing in the affected ear
- nausea, vomiting, and sweating caused by severe vertigo
- tinnitus, or the sense of ringing, in the affected ear
- vertigo, with attacks lasting anywhere from a few minutes to 24 hours

Anyone with Meniere's disease will experience at least two to three of the following symptoms at one time:

- aural fullness
- hearing loss
- tinnitus
- vertigo

Most people with Meniere's disease do not experience symptoms between episodes. So, many of these symptoms could be caused by other problems in the ear if they occur during a period without an attack. Meniere's disease can also be confused with another inner ear disorder, labyrinthitis.

A typical attack or episode of Meniere's is preceded by fullness in one ear. Auditory fluctuation or changes in tinnitus may also precede an attack. A Meniere's attack generally involves vertigo, imbalance, nausea and vomiting, and acute hearing reduction. After a **severe attack,** most people feel exhausted and sleep for several hours. There is a significant amount of inconsistency in the duration of symptoms, with a few people experiencing **brief shocks** and others having constant unsteadiness. An unusual variant is an **invisible hand,** where individuals feel as if they are being pushed over. High sensitivity to visual stimuli is common. During the attack, the eyes jump (nystagmus).

In most cases, gradual hearing loss occurs in the affected ear(s). A low-frequency sensorineural pattern is initially heard, but it usually changes into either a flat loss or a peaked pattern as time goes on. Although an acute attack can be incapacitating, Meniere's disease is not fatal.

Additional Symptoms of Meniere's Disease

When dealing with Meniere's, several other symptoms may be present besides the four primary symptoms (Vertigo, Hearing loss, Tinnitus, and Aural fullness). These include:

- **Brain fog** - dedicating a tremendous amount of energy to maintain equilibrium and stay fast takes a toll on activities such as recalling details or short-term memory. Thinking might become slow.

- **Cognitive issues** - memory difficulties and concentration problems link everything from fibromyalgia to post-concussion syndrome.

- **Fatigue** - a common problem for those with chronic fatigue syndrome of fibromyalgia.

- **Nausea** - feeling as if you want to throw up all the time.

- **Psychological changes** - due to the unpredictable nature of symptoms and the chronic nature of the disorder, people with vestibular system problems tend to suffer from anxiety and depression.

- **Sensitivity to light and sound** - are common migraine symptoms.

- **Vision impairment** - the link between the vestibular system and vision is apparent to people with Meniere's, and the potential for vision correction, including glasses and contacts, should be explored.

You may have observed the connection between Meniere's and several other chronic health disorders from the above. The factor that ties these symptoms together begins with a head or neck trauma.

The Upper Cervical Solution for Meniere's and Vertigo

Meniere's disease and its many symptoms like vertigo correlate to a misalignment of the atlas (the top bone in the spine). The atlas plays a crucial role in everything from brainstem function to facilitating vertebral artery flow. Obtaining the proper amount of blood to the ears is essential in the vestibular system's operation (which controls balance). Also, the appropriate function of the Eustachian tubes can be affected by long-term neck issues.

Upper cervical chiropractic focuses on the gentle and accurate adjustment of the atlas. As soon as this vital vertebra is in the proper position, the body has a chance to heal. Blood may flow to where it needs to go, and the atlas again protects the brainstem.

Damage Caused By Meniere's Disease

The following problems are damages caused by Meniere's:

- **Hair cell death** - repeated attacks of Meniere's kills hair cells in the inner ear. This process occurring over the years frequently results in functional deafness. Cochlear (hearing) hair cells are most sensitive, with vestibular hair cells being more resilient. There is a slow decline in the caloric response in the diseased ear over roughly 15 years.

- **Mechanical changes to the ear** - disruption of the inner ear is probable, with dilation of the utricle and saccule of the ear. The saccule may dilate so that it is adherent to the underside of the stapes footplate in later stages. This mechanical disruption and distortion of the natural inner ear structure may gradually onset chronic unsteadiness. Recurring dilation and shrinkage of the utricle also explain occasional episodes of another internal ear disorder called benign paroxysmal positional vertigo (BPPV). Lastly, there may be a rupture of the suspensory system for the membranous labyrinth related to vestibular atelectasis. This could create some mechanical instability of the utricle and saccule and consequently some chronic unsteadiness.

Part 3   DIAGNOSING MENIERE'S DISEASE

If experiencing symptoms of Meniere's disease, see a doctor immediately. Your doctor will order tests that will scrutinize your balance and hearing and then rule out other causes of your symptoms.

What Type Of Doctor Diagnoses Meniere's?

The **Ear, Nose, and Throat (ENT) Doctor** (Otolaryngologist) is the point person for diagnosing Meniere's Disease. When a **Primary Physician** cannot alleviate the pain and suffering of their patient, and they suspect Meniere's, they will refer them to an ENT for verification and then treatment. This doctor will review medical history details and then ask questions about reaction and symptom experiences. They will then measure that information against the criteria utilized to diagnose Meniere's.

Testing For Meniere's Disease

If the results are potentially positive, the doctor may request a hearing test to establish a baseline for any hearing loss. The doctor may order the following procedures to find the cause of your symptoms:

- **A hearing test** - or audiometry is used to determine if you are experiencing hearing loss. In this test, you put on headphones and hear noises of various pitches and volumes. You must indicate when you can and cannot hear a tone, so the technician can determine if you suffer from hearing loss. Your hearing will be tested to determine if you can distinguish between similar sounds. In this test segment, you will listen to words through the headphones and repeat what you hear. The test will tell the doctor if you have a hearing problem in one or both ears.

    A problem in the inner ear or a nerve in the ear can cause hearing loss. Electrocochleography (ECog) testing will gauge electrical activity in the inner ear. An auditory brainstem response (ABR) test verifies the function of the hearing nerves and the hearing center in the brain. These tests will inform your doctor if the problem is caused by the inner ear or a nerve in the ear.

- **Balance tests** - are performed to test the function of the inner ear. In having Meniere's, you will have a reduced balance response in one or both ear(s). The balance test most used for Meniere's disease is

electronystagmography (ENG). Here electrodes are placed around your eyes to detect eye movement since the balance response in the inner ear causes eye movements. Warm and cold water is pushed into the ear during this test. The water causes the balance function to work, and involuntary eye movements will be tracked. Any abnormalities will indicate a problem with the inner ear.
- Today, rotary chair testing is used less often. It shows the doctor whether your problem is caused by an ear or brain issue. When used in addition to ENG testing, the ENG results can be incorrect if you have ear damage or wax blocking one of your ear's canals. Your eye movements are carefully recorded in this test while the chair moves.
- Vestibular-evoked myogenic potential (VEMP) testing is used to measure sound sensitivity of the vestibule of the inner ear, and posturography testing helps determine what part of your balance system is not functioning correctly. You will react to various balance challenges while wearing a safety harness and standing barefoot.

- **Other tests** - issues with the brain, such as multiple sclerosis (MS) or brain tumors, can cause symptoms similar to Meniere's. Your doctor can ask for tests to rule out these and other conditions. They may also request a head MRI or a cranial CT scan to assess likely brain problems.

Part 4   TREATMENT OF MENIERE'S DISEASE

Although Meniere's is a chronic condition with no cure, various treatments can help with its' symptoms, from medications to surgery in the most severe cases.

Noninvasive Therapies And Procedures
- **Medication** - your doctor may prescribe medication to help with symptoms of the disease. Medicines for motion sickness can relieve the symptoms of vertigo, nausea, and vomiting (meclizine or diazepam). If nausea and vomiting become a problem, your doctor may prescribe an antiemetic or anti-nausea medication (promethazine). Diuretics are long-term medications used to reduce fluid retention.
  Note: a problem with fluid in the inner ear is believed to cause Meniere's disease. If it happens, your doctor may prescribe a diuretic to help reduce the amount of fluid in your body. Your doctor may also inject medication into your inner ear through the middle ear to help reduce vertigo symptoms.

- **Physical therapy** - vestibular rehabilitation exercises can improve symptoms of vertigo. These exercises help train your brain to account for the difference in balance between your ears. A physical therapist can teach you these exercises.

- **Hearing aids** - an audiologist can treat hearing loss, usually by fitting you with a hearing aid.

Aggressive Procedures
If the conservative treatments listed above are unsuccessful, your doctor might recommend more aggressive treatment.

- **Middle ear injections** - are for medications injected into and then absorbed into the inner ear to improve vertigo symptoms. Such treatment is done in the doctor's office. Available injections include:
    - Gentamicin, an antibiotic that is toxic to your inner ear. It reduces the balancing function of the ear, with your other ear assuming responsibility for balance. However, there is a risk of this antibiotic creating further hearing loss.

- o Steroids, such as dexamethasone may help control some vertigo attacks. Although dexamethasone might be slightly less effective than gentamicin, it is less likely to cause further hearing loss.

- **Surgery** - if vertigo attacks associated with Meniere's disease are severe and debilitating with other treatments not helping, surgery might be an option. Procedures may include:
  - o **Endolymphatic sac procedure** - the endolymphatic sac plays a role in regulating inner ear fluid levels. The endolymphatic sac is decompressed throughout the procedure, relieving excess fluid levels. In some instances, this procedure is coupled with the placement of a shunt, a tube that drains excess fluid from the inner ear.
  - o **Labyrinthectomy** - in this procedure, the surgeon removes the *balance portion* of the inner ear, thereby eliminating both balance and hearing function by the affected ear. This procedure is done only if you have near-total or total hearing loss in the affected ear.
  - o **Vestibular nerve section** - a procedure that involves cutting the nerve that links *balance and movement sensors* (vestibular nerve) in the inner ear to the brain. This procedure typically corrects problems with vertigo while attempting to preserve hearing in the affected ear. It does require general anesthesia and an overnight hospital stay.

Part 5   DIET and MENIERE'S

Diet Goals
Because of Meniere's unique etiology (cause) and prognosis, **'diet is crucial in managing the disease.'** The diet focuses on reducing the frequency and intensity of the episodic symptoms the disease causes. Meniere's disease is closely linked to and dependent upon the body's blood system and fluid balances. Specific dietary changes will help with managing the disease's conditions effectively.

The first goal of the diet is to rid the body of substances that cause and stimulate water retention. Water retention worsens the symptoms because excess fluid can build up within the ear. Another goal of the diet is to decrease overall fluid volumes through natural diuretics. Overall, body fluids reduction can reduce fluid buildup in the inner ear. Eliminating substances that cause constriction of regular blood flow and limiting the use of dietary substances are additional areas the diet emphasizes.

The Diet
People on this diet should avoid foods and drinks high in sugar and salt. Sugar intake stimulates the body to respond with insulin, and insulin retains sodium. Then sodium triggers the body to keep more water. The following guide will help you in resolving this cycle:

Food and drink to avoid - think about balance, tinnitus, and nausea when choosing foods to avoid. Eliminate foods and beverages that exasperate the above symptoms and replace them with suitable alternatives for your overall well-being. This process consists of five basic steps.

1. **Avoid caffeine** - it is a stimulant that can exasperate Meniere's symptoms. Likewise, limit alcohol consumption to a maximum of one glass a day. Consumption of more than this may trigger a migraine or dizziness.

2. **Avoid foods high in sodium and carbohydrates** - salt intake increases the body's water weight retention, which increases inner ear fluid pressure. This creates an ideal environment for a Meniere's attack. Canned and processed food has a lot of salt. In terms of carbohydrates (bread, pasta), these can also increase water retention. This is why people who follow low-carb diets lose weight quickly at first. Those pounds are water released from the body. In either case, you can add

potassium-rich foods into your diet instead. This will act as a diuretic and can even offset a meal where you accidentally overate salt. Additional natural diuretics include dandelion tea (do not consume before bed), hibiscus, ginger, nettle, beets, asparagus, and celery.

3. **Avoid MSG** - some people find that it triggers their Meniere's symptoms. On the list of what not to eat, avoid MSG. Additionally, do not consume plant protein extracts, yeast extracts, textured protein, corn oil, malt extract or flavoring, broth or stock, seasonings like beef or chicken, soy, or whey protein concentrate.
Note: Aspartame (NutraSweet, Equal) creates Meniere-like symptoms in some people. It is also a contributor to depression.

4. Balance your meals throughout the day and ensure continuity throughout the week. It means eating consistent proportions at the same time every day. Do not skip meals.

5. Remain hydrated using water or other liquids so long as they do not have a lot of sugar.

Avoiding Sugar and Salt - research indicates that salt and sugar are at the top of the list of what to avoid if you have Meniere's disease. Major offenders among **simple sugars** are:

- candy including chocolate
- galactose (found in dairy foods)
- high Fructose Corn Syrup
- honey
- jams and jellies
- maltose (in molasses)
- soda
- table sugar

From the perspective of **salt intake,** people with Meniere's Disease should limit themselves to 1,500 mg of sodium daily. More than that will increase water weight. Following is the list of foods that have high levels of salt and alternatives for the diet:

- **Breads and Grains** - avoid salted rolls, quick breads, pancake mix, pizza, salted crackers, instant potatoes, and stuffing. Alternatives include muffins, rice, pasta, low-sodium crackers, unsalted pretzels, and chips.

- **Condiments and Fats** - avoid soy sauce, marinades, bottled salad dressing, salted butter, ketchup, and mustard. Alternatives include vegetable oil, unsalted oil, vinegar, low-sodium salad dressings, or sauces.

- **Dairy** - avoid buttermilk, processed cheese (or cheese spreads), cheese sauce, and cottage cheese. Instead, eat ice milk, cream cheese, and mozzarella.

- **Eggs, Fish, Meat, and Poultry** - avoid smoked, salted, and cured meat. The same holds for fish and poultry items like ham, hot dogs, sardines, cold cuts, and anchovies. Alternatives include fresh frozen pork, beef, and oil or water-packed poultry and fish.

- **Fruit and Vegetables** - canned vegetables and vegetable juices, olives, pickles, packaged mixes like au gratin potatoes, pre-prepared salsa. Alternatives include fresh potatoes or frozen fries, low-sodium vegetable juice, fresh or frozen fruit juice, dried fruit, and plain frozen vegetables.

High Sodium Foods - almost all canned food contains salt as a flavoring or preservative. Of particular note to avoid are the following:

- Beverages - vegetable juice, sports drinks
- Cheese - almost every type
- Condiments - Worcestershire, soy, salad dressing (including mixes), ketchup, and sweet relish
- Frozen Dinners - all types
- Ice Cream - brands with add-ins like cookie bits
- Packaged Food - including breakfast cereals, macaroni & cheese, and flavored rice
- Packaged Mixes - cakes, brownies, and bread
- Pickled Items - including olives and sauerkraut
- Processed Meat - including bacon, sausage, ham, and salami
- Snacks - the snack aisle in the grocery store has a majority of what is brimming with salt
- Spices - garlic or onion salt (get powder instead). Bouillon cubes, malt extract, spice blends

Individual ingredients to avoid - specific components affect Meniere's symptoms more than others. It would be best if you avoid edibles that trigger migraines specifically, such as those items having tyramine, an amino acid. Examples include bananas, brie, cheddar cheese, chicken livers, chocolate, figs, nuts, red wine, smoked meat, and yogurt.

The above impacts fluid regulation in the body, including blood flow. They may also cause vertigo, headaches, and other Meniere manifestations.

Food And Drink To Consume

The best foods and beverages to consume are limited simple sugars and low sodium.

- Foods that contain complex sugars instead of simple sugars that are safe to eat are:
    - raw nuts, fresh beans, lentils, whole grains, sweet potatoes, and brown rice

- Foods and beverages known to be natural diuretics that will help reduce fluid retention. Natural diuretics include:
    - fresh asparagus, ginger, beets, fresh watermelon, fresh lemons, nettle leaves, cucumbers, fresh mint leaves, fresh peaches, fresh pineapple, and cilantro leaves

- Whenever someone eats food, they should consume an equal amount of water or other caffeine-free fluids. Having an equal distribution of food and fluids helps manage inner ear fluid levels. For symptom reduction, eat:
    - dark leafy greens like kale, spinach, cabbage, collard greens, broccoli, plantain, arugula, chard, and turnip greens

Effectiveness Of The Diet

The disease is dependent upon fluid levels and balance in the body, and the diet is based on foods and beverages that manipulate the fluid levels to reduce symptoms of the disease.

Note: fluid levels can change rapidly, so a deviation from the diet can worsen symptoms. It is also reported that Meniere's disease diet works better when allergies and food sensitivities are avoided, such as gluten and lactose. Some caffeine medications can also be problematic since the diet states caffeine should not be consumed. Finally, a person needs to anticipate the loss of fluids related to exposure to heat and physical activities and attempt to replace them before they deplete.

Part 6   **VITAMINS, MEDICATIONS, and HERBALS**

There are many vitamins and supplements available without a prescription (OTC). We do not advocate starting on a regimen of supplements without first consulting the physician monitoring your Meniere's. Use the following information as a **'talking point'** to ascertain the best care plan for your symptom specifics.

Antihistamines/Anti-Allergy Preparations - products like meclizine or diazepam can help for sickness, often caused by vertigo, nausea, and vomiting attacks.

B Vitamins - B12 sometimes reduces ringing in the ears. Many people who experience tinnitus with hearing loss exhibit B12 deficiencies. While the exact reason B12 appears to work is unknown, there seems to be a tie between this vitamin and healthy nerve functions. Studies indicate that Vitamin B1 (Thiamine) and B3 (Niacin) might decrease Meniere's symptoms while improving overall energy.

CBD Oil - is a non-psychoactive cannabinoid that comes from marijuana. Many studies show that CBD has various medical applications, including anti-nausea and anti-inflammatory substances. Beyond this, it may relieve some of the stress that Meniere's symptoms cause.

Charcoal Capsules - activated charcoal capsules appear to clear out **'brain fog'** that people with Meniere experience, especially after an attack. It must be used with moderation as it has a high salt content. It also has the capacity for absorbing other prescription medications.

Dandelion Root Capsules - a natural diuretic that keeps you from water retention. Many people find it easier to take a capsule than eat dandelion greens or flowers.

Essential Oils - are oils that some people find helpful with dizziness and vertigo. The most prevalent components in these blends are natural Birch, Lavender, Ylang-Ylang, Peppermint, Frankincense, Chamomile, and Myrrh. Other potential essentials for Meniere's light headedness include:

- Basil Oil
- Bergamot Oil
- Clary-Sage Oil
- Cypress Oil
- Ginger Oil

- Lemon Balm Oil
- Neroli Oil
- Rose Oil
- Rosemary Oil
- Tangerine Oil

Sample a little dab behind each ear when you feel dizzy or nauseous.

Ginkgo Biloba - is a natural supplement that decreases blood viscosity (thickness). This may improve blood flow to the brain and inner ear, reducing tinnitus.

Tinnitus Formulas - the formulas on the market typically have one or more central ingredients (ginkgo Biloba, zinc, garlic, Lemon Bioflavonoids, or Lipo-Flavonoids). These ingredients target the inner ear function and blood flow. Lemon bioflavonoids have the added benefit of having antioxidant qualities. It is stated that the preceding can take upwards of three months to see any measurable results.

Vitamin C and D3 - these two vitamins are essential, particularly for overall well-being. Vitamin D deficiency can increase Meniere's depression. Vitamin C is a broad tonic-like antioxidant.

Over the Counter (OTC) Medications

Some over-the-counter medications can trigger and worsen existing vestibular problems. Watch and track your reaction to:

- antacids
- aspirin
- ibuprofen
- smoking cessation products

Herbal Treatment Options

Alfalfa - improves overall cardiovascular health and contains essential minerals like iron, zinc, and magnesium.

Alpha Lipoic Acid - targets Meniere's progressive hearing loss. Herbs are not the best source for this supplement, but you can try spinach, peas, and tomatoes.

Calcium - supports the bones in your inner ear. Herbs that contain calcium include savory, dill, oregano, mint, sage, celery seed, and parsley.

Chromium Picolinate - moderates blood sugars. High or low blood sugar often leads to Meniere-like vertigo. Herbs that contain this element include yarrow, nettle, catnip, and wild yam.

CoQ10 - recommended for improved circulation and oxygen use. Parsley is the go-to herb for this supplement.

Dandelion - is a natural diuretic that may help keep the levels of the inner ear fluids more stable for Meniere's patients. It can be consumed as tea. *Warning: those with ragweed allergies may also have a sensitivity to dandelion.* If so, you might try black caraway, hibiscus tea, ginger, and parsley.

Echinacea - since Meniere's may have links to autoimmune disorders, echinacea boosts the immune system.

Ginseng - for motion sickness symptoms that occur with vertigo.

Lipase enzyme - some people find this supplement helps with dizziness. Oats contain this enzyme.

Lysine - plays many roles in the body, including connective tissue repair, helping absorb calcium, and reducing anxiety. Herbs containing Lysine are lavender, rosemary, amaranth, and basil.

Mint - a good source of Lysine. Some Meniere's patients use this as an herbal treatment for nausea in tea form.

MSM - is a sulfur compound that some say heals damaged tissues and offsets allergies. Herbs other than garlic are not high in MSM, but you can get sulfur from foods like kale, cabbage, broccoli, turnips, and onions.

Niacin (also called Vitamin B3) - improves blood circulation. The top five herbs for Niacin are paprika, ginger, red pepper, fennel, and sage. These have at least 25% of the recommended daily intake for Vitamin B3, with paprika having twice that.

Noni - used in juice form, this fruit seems to help with hearing loss (it's very sour).

Vinpocetine - increases blood flow to the inner ear, which may offset vertigo. It comes from the Periwinkle plant, but it is easiest to find in commercially prepared products.

Vitamin B12 - used for tinnitus. Herbal treatment options include alfalfa, dandelion, and hops.

Vitamin C - this antioxidant fights inflammation. Some of the best culinary herbs with high levels of vitamin C are parsley, chives, basil, and thyme.

Wheatgrass - rich in protein and amino acids, wheatgrass can boost your immunity.

MENIERE'S DISEASE – What is Meniere's, Symptoms, Treatment, and Lifestyle

Part 7   LIFESTYLE CHANGES

In addition to dietary changes, the following lifestyle changes may help:

- managing stress and anxiety through psychotherapy or medication
- regularly eating, to help regulate fluids in the body
- resting during vertigo attacks

It is crucial to quit smoking and avoid any allergens since both make the symptoms of Meniere's disease worse. Statistics indicate that 70% of smokers have increased hearing loss over those who do not smoke. Chemicals in cigarettes constrict blood vessels, including vessels in the ears. Nicotine alone can bring on dizziness and tinnitus. Smoking cessation is prudent since results are also symptoms of Meniere's.

Safety
Consider implementing the following safety measures:

- avoid driving; find a car-buddy
- avoid reaching upward toward high items, and avoid heights if possible
- educate your family, friends, and coworkers on Meniere's symptoms and what to do when you have an episode
- use sensible shoes with flat bottoms and good traction

Home Style
Go through your living space and implement the following measures:

- if no standard handholds are available, put grab bars in the shower, near the toilet, and on stairways
- replace throw rugs with mats having a non-skid backing
- add night lights with automatic activation for safe walking when it's dark
- get a step stool with handrails
- move shoes, dog toys, and other small items out of common walkways to prevent falls

Managing An Attack
During an acute attack, lay down on a firm surface. Stay motionless with eyes open and fixed on a stationary object. Do not drink or sip water, as you will most likely vomit. Stay in this position until the spinning passes, then get up

SLOWLY. After the attack subsides, you will probably feel exhausted and need to sleep for several hours.

If vomiting persists and you cannot take fluids for longer than 24 hours (12 hours for children), contact your doctor. They can prescribe nausea medication or vestibular suppressant medication. They may want to see you or even admit you to the hospital if you are dehydrated. Meclizine (Antivert), lorazepam, and clonazepam are frequently used vestibular suppressant medications, and Compazine, Phenergan, or Ondansetron are widely used drugs for nausea.

Part 8   MISCELLANEOUS SUGGESTIONS

Environmental Support
Two things that you can control in your home are light and sound. Bright lights often bother people with Meniere's, as do sharp or loud sounds, which may trigger an episode. If you sense a headache coming on or are starting to feel shaky, turn down the lights and put on relaxing music or nature sounds for relaxation. Additionally, because you are dealing with dizziness, look around to verify that you are safe if you experience a Meniere's drop attack.

Stress and Sleep
Nothing is worse for our bodies, minds, and spirit than stress. People living with Meniere often experience stress and anxiety over the unpredictable nature of their vertigo attacks. That means avoiding stressors is vital to be at your best ability. Doing this will lower your risk for other problems like heart disorders and poor digestion.

Sleep helps reduce stress. If you do not get good sleep, your anxiety levels increase, and you feel on edge. Maintain a good quality daily sleep routine. If you have trouble sleeping, try herbs that help relax and calm. Enjoy chamomile, valerian, lavender, or lemon balm tea. Read the label to verify that you are getting a non-caffeinated product.

Support
Anyone who has a chronic illness would benefit from a solid support system. What this means is educating your family and friends about Meniere's Disease. They will need to know how to help when you have an attack, keeping you safe and comfortable. Create a plan that they can use as a guide for their reference.

Travel
People who have Meniere's might have a challenging time with travel. Sometimes, they will feel like they are moving even after the vehicle stops. Things can be done for Meniere's symptoms triggered by traveling.

- **Preparing for Flight** - if you are flying, avoid seats near the engines and try to book an aisle seat to navigate to the lavatory with ease. Most airlines will accommodate these requests if you explain your condition. Also, talk to your physician about steps to prepare for the pressure-changing effects in your ears (such as earplugs to relieve your ear discomfort, clogging, and popping via naturally filtering and regulating air pressure). Additionally, bring chewing gum with you, and swallowing often will help to regulate ear pressure.

- **Public Transportation** - if you are on a bus or subway, make sure you are seated. The best thing to do is to seat yourself before movement begins. Once in motion, it can throw you off balance, and you risk falling.

- **Transport by Boat** - when voyaging by sea, you can expect to face issues with balance until you get your **'sea legs.'** Try and book a room mid-ship where the moving sensation lessens. When you are on the deck, look out toward a fixed point on the horizon so your eyes do not see as much movement. If you get sick, stay hydrated.

- **Vehicle** - if going by car, it is best to have another person drive for you. If this is not possible, take someone along for the ride who understands your conditions and symptoms. Ensure the person knows what to do about a vertigo attack when it occurs.

Note: with all forms of travel, remember to pack the medications prescribed by your doctor or carry an over-the-counter medicine with you to control Meniere's symptoms! Nothing is more frustrating than getting a pharmacy to approve necessary items for an out-of-town situation.

Part 9   CAREGIVERS MANAGEMENT

Meniere's caregivers have common issues that they face. Meniere's does not just affect the sufferer. It also impacts family, friends, and coworkers. Meniere constraints also create challenges inside and outside the home.

To help the caregiver understand the disease, we have included the following:

Let us begin by explaining what the disease feels like ………. Meniere's Disease starts with problems in the inner ear. Typically, only one ear is affected. The result of having a Meniere's attack is feeling like the whole world is spinning like a toy top. If you can, remember when you were a child and twirled around until you fell? People with Meniere's often have that feeling, supplemented by ringing in the ear (Tinnitus) and sometimes feeling like the ear is packed with something causing pressure.

Vertigo Episodes
This is one of the acute symptoms of Meniere's Disease. The affected may be sitting perfectly still and feel dizzy. Alternatively, the feeling makes you feel off-center as if you are moving when you are not. These spells come and go and vary in duration.

To understand Vertigo, you need to know about the ears. Sound travels to the eardrum via the ear canal. The bones in the inner ear act as the brain's translators, turning sound into a vibration that travels to the brain. Everything in the inner ear is susceptible to immediate feedback about the sound.

Some types of vertigo start in the spinal cord or brain. Meniere's vertigo is considered peripheral because the inner ear experiences fluid build-up. Specific instances of Meniere's-related vertigo begin with body movements such as rolling over in bed, standing up quickly, or just tilting your head. These movements can make you feel faint and can also result in nausea. If someone were to examine you at that time, your eyes could be abnormally moving.

Note: when vertigo accompanies weakness, disorientation, or lateral signs of coordination loss, this symptom may signify a stroke instead of Meniere's disease presenting itself.

Hearing Loss

Another Meniere's disease symptom is loss of hearing. At the start of Meniere's, your hearing aptitude may change, some days good and others worse. Hearing loss can become permanent over time. People with Meniere's state their ears feel plugged, and sounds are fuzzy or off, and some also experience sound sensitivity. The difference between hearing in the two ears creates mismatched brain signals resulting in distortion. So, it becomes difficult for the person living with Meniere to listen to things properly, particularly in a noisy space. Additionally, loud noises can become uncomfortable.

When you have just one good ear, you cannot always determine the direction of a sound. Since your other ear has some loss, you always feel like sounds are coming from the other side. To make matters worse, sufferers tend to turn their head so that their good ear faces the discussion or situation, resulting in neck stiffness or soreness.

Tinnitus (Ringing in the Ear)

Tinnitus is a common occurrence, affecting millions in the United States alone. It is challenging to describe Tinnitus, no matter the cause. Some experience it as a steady sound, like one extended radio frequency that never disappears. Others hear:

- a hum or buzz
- a musical note
- chirping like crickets
- clicking
- hissing
- roaring like waves or wind
- screeching
- static
- trills or whistling

Some hear a combination of these sounds. Tinnitus can be continuous or intermittent and differs in loudness. Some find it more apparent when rooms are quiet. Consequently, some people will lose concentration or experience insomnia.

Tinnitus has a connection to hearing loss, but it does not cause the loss. It also impacts sound sensitivity, where a person reacts badly to specific types of noise. And, like many other physical issues, it may have a wide variety of causes other than Meniere's disease. These causes include:

- aging: as we age, the inner ear may experience deterioration
- auditory nerve tumor

- autoimmune diseases
- circulatory issues or anemia
- diabetes
- ear infections
- ear wax buildup
- head or neck injury
- long term exposure to loud sounds (a most common cause that also impacts hearing loss)
- medication side effects (drugs including antidepressants, sedatives, and antibiotics all have this potential)
- The temporomandibular joint (TMJ) is a condition of the jaw
- under-active thyroid

Alcohol, caffeine, and smoking may make Tinnitus worse.

Stuffy or Full Ear
With Meniere's, there can be times when you feel pressure in your affected ear, similar to being in an airplane or being underwater. This can be very uncomfortable, especially when accompanied by other Meniere's symptoms like vertigo and tinnitus.

Other conditions besides Meniere's can cause ear pressure. Some of the most common causes include:

- a cold
- allergies
- an ear infection
- ear wax buildup

Please consult your primary physician to rule out these problems or diagnose them and provide a care plan for relief.

Nausea and Vomiting
Feeling sick is not unusual for people experiencing a bout of Meniere's vertigo. Once these attacks come on, the longer they last, the more likely you may feel like you have the flu. Some doctors suggest keeping over-the-counter motion sickness medications on hand.

In some harsh moments, you might even have diarrhea. This, combined with vomiting, is why physicians recommend that people living with Meniere's remain hydrated.

Unusual Eye Motion
While in a Meniere's episode, some have odd, rapid eye movements. It may just be one eye or both resulting in blurry vision. Generally, the eyes move side to side, increasing the vertigo feelings.

Drop Attacks
As the name implies, this Meniere disease symptom brings a person to the floor. This is known as Tumarkin's otolithic crisis. Most drop attacks occur in the later stages of Meniere's. A drop attack makes you feel like someone pushed you forcefully, resulting in a fall. This pushing sensation goes away quickly, and you do not lose consciousness, but your balance may remain off after that.

Cold Sweats and Weariness
If you have ever had hot or cold flashes, you understand how people living with Meniere's feel during some episodes. Vertigo seems to set it off, so your physician may prescribe medicine that helps alleviate dizziness.

Beyond that, Meniere's disease impacts a person's energy level considerably. That same fatigue may cause some flare-ups, meaning that the sufferer should concentrate on getting enough rest and not over-extending themselves.

Moodiness
There is no doubt that any chronic disease impacts mental health. Meniere's disease is no exception. Suffers report their Meniere's disease symptoms as mood changers, especially before episodes. There is also anxiety, wondering when the next attack may come. At the same time, Meniere's disease may not be the root of mood changes. It is something to remain aware of and potentially seek out counseling or other aid.

Migraines
Usually are not discussed in Meniere's, but they can undoubtedly be a symptom. Yes, diet and lifestyle contribute to severe headaches, but people with Meniere's sometimes get migraines during an episode.

AFTERWORD

Thank you for reading,

**MENIERE'S DISEASE
What is Meniere's,
Symptoms, Treatment, and Lifestyle**

We hope you enjoyed this Life-Health Media USA Publication

Thank you again, valued reader,
and we hope to meet you again on another book.

ABOUT THE AUTHOR

Pierre Mouchette is the Founder and CEO of Real Property Experts LLC. He is a graduate of New York University, with a Master's in Business Administration, a Certificate in Real Estate Law - Fairfield University - CT, a Graduate of the Realtors Institute - CT, and held licensing as a Real Estate Broker, and a Mortgage Broker.

Pierre is currently authoring Books, Booklets, How-to-Articles, and Guides in retirement. Pierre has an extensive background in real estate investment, business management, and sales, supplemented by decades of hands-on experience in building systems engineering, development, evaluation, and various analytical engineering studies.

Pierre launched Real Property Experts in 2013 to simplify real estate investing by connecting investors through innovative technology using background knowledge and experience. In 2018, Pierre created THE SYNCHRONICITY INVESTOR (TSI), a real estate website to facilitate world-class solutions for real estate investors and investment businesses.

During the winter of 2021, Pierre created **Enviro | Life Publications** to bring Environmental and Life Knowledge to a growing TSI audience. Exploring the Internet and using all sources available, this entity will bring to our audience through its Research, Information that is Transparent and easy to understand, thereby making them more Knowledgeable.

Life-Health Media USA

- presents -

An Enviro | Life Knowledge Publications

LIFE HEALTH

DISEASES
 MENIER'S DISEASE – What Is Meniere's, Symptoms, Treatment, and Lifestyle

HEALTH
 OVERACTIVE BLADDER – Symptoms, Treatments, and Lifestyle Remedies

Made in the USA
Columbia, SC
02 April 2022

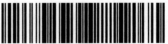